YOU ARE WORTH YOUR HEALTH

Introducing 360 Living

YOU ARE WORTH YOUR HEALTH

Introducing 360 Living

Carmen Keith, MD

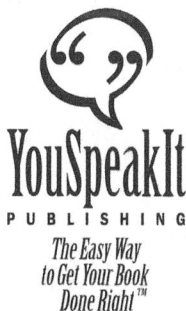

YouSpeakIt

PUBLISHING

*The Easy Way
to Get Your Book
Done Right*™

www.YouSpeakItPublishing.com

ISBN: 978-1-945446-43-6

I would like to dedicate this book to you, my dear reader, to your best self, whom you have envisioned but perhaps found too difficult to achieve. I would also like to dedicate this to my great-grandmother, Ma, who taught me the importance of self-provision and hard work, speaking my mind, and above all else, loving others.

Acknowledgments

I would first like to acknowledge my family—my husband, Josh, and my three children Noah, Josie, and Elijah—for supporting Mom through this process and for being very patient as I wrote my first book.

To my parents, for giving me their full support throughout my life, for being the wind under my wings, and for encouraging me to do what no one else would even attempt.

To my Ethel, because you know who you are, and every Lucy needs her Ethel.

To the many mentors whom I've known throughout the years; some of you know me and, frankly, some of you do not. You have all been so encouraging and a powerful influence on my journey to become the healer that I am called to be. I hope that in the future we may meet.

I would also like to acknowledge my fur baby, Harvey the Cat. Without Harvey's companionship, it would have been much more difficult to write this book. His purring kept me grounded.

To God, my Creator, my Sustainer—without your influence in my life none of this would be possible. Thank you for getting me out of my comfort zone.

Finally, I would like to acknowledge the You Speak It team, especially Sunny Sukumar. I could not have done this without Sunny, and also Keith and Maura Leon, who showed me that I could write a book. I always wanted to write, but thought the task would be too daunting. Thank you for making this possible.

Contents

Foreword

I first met Carmen on an elevator in Atlanta, Georgia. We were the only two on the elevator and rather than ignore each other, we began what turned out to be a serendipitous conversation that was the beginning of a beautiful relationship — both professionally and personally.

Carmen was living in the world of modern medicine, frustrated by a desire to help people be well in a system that supports sickness. She believed it possible to move medicine in a better direction, and in her quest to find that path, she found functional medicine. Carmen will tell you that functional medicine is everything a patient expects medicine to be, and I agree with her.

What she will not tell you is that she brings something to her patients that cannot be taught in any school or learned at any conference. Carmen brings passion and positive energy into every encounter. When she opens her mouth, her compassion and love for people overflow. In my forty-five years of medical practice, I have not met anyone who is a better physician than Carmen. Just knowing her has made me better too. I believe it is this passion, blended with her tender heart, that allowed her to walk away from a prestigious job in the world of modern medicine and embark on a path to help people find true health and wellness.

Carmen is a brilliant physician whose insight into the current healthcare system is both enlightening and frightening. She sees its crumbling foundation and addresses honestly and fearlessly the necessity for change. She wants to help as many people as possible find a different way, a better way, a caring way to embrace the healthy life they desire. Spend just five minutes with her, and you will know you have met the person who has both the knowledge and heart to help you fulfill your health destiny.

As you read, *You Are Worth Your Health,* I believe you will find the same kindhearted and enthusiastic physician I did on that elevator several years ago. Her positive energy is irresistible. Feel her heartbeat as you read each page, knowing that her deepest desire is for you to finish the book empowered to change your life. Please, don't just read the book and then set it aside and walk away. Honor my friend, my brilliant colleague, my heartmate, Carmen, by pursuing the life of health and wellness you were created for!

Guy O. Danielson, MD
Board-Certified Neurosurgeon
Founder of Integrative Health Matters
Trailblazer in Functional and
Regenerative Medicine

Introduction

Our healthcare system isn't working. This book is about the current challenges we face as a nation and, more importantly, it's about a better way, a different way, to achieve the health that you deserve.

I am a Harvard-trained physician who, through my own health crisis, found that the current healthcare system was unable to provide me with long-lasting health and wellness. I began my journey to find what this health really looked like, and I realized that as I discovered answers, I could not keep them to myself. I had a moral and ethical responsibility as a physician to share those with you. As I will also share, my professional health was also in jeopardy. I had to embrace a different way. My practice is now about prevention and lifestyle as well as treating existing conditions through root-cause analysis. This book offers a look into what that means.

Read the book from start to finish with a mind open to the possibility that *healthcare* may not be an accurate term to describe the system that promotes itself as caring for us. Imagine there is the possibility that there are other methods that can create lasting health and vitality to enable you to thrive in the life that you have been given.

I hope that you will come to understand that you are worthy of good health. I hope you will begin to question how your life is now, and if it is where you want it to be.

Are you now living the life you envisioned when you were younger?

Where did you imagine yourself to be at the age you are now?

If you are not where you thought you would be, I hope this book inspires you to take the first steps toward the life you have always dreamed of.

CHAPTER ONE

Our Healthcare Crisis

OUR RELIANCE ON HEALTHCARE

What is the foundation of our national healthcare system, and why is it in crisis?

I want to begin by explaining why the current system of healthcare is fallible, and why, despite its problems, we continue to rely heavily on it.

We have to understand where healthcare came from and the direction in which it is currently heading. Despite the exorbitant costs to us, our health continues to decline. Your expectations of the healthcare system creating health are being eroded by less time with your physician and more pills in your medication box.

Does this resound with you?

Let's take a closer look.

The Beginnings of Our Healthcare System

Doctors originally played an important role in the community. They paid house calls to their patients in both emergency situations and for more routine needs, such as delivering babies and tending to the ill and the elderly.

Physicians have historically been called upon for their skills in acute healthcare. As more illness has emerged and the burden of chronic disease has increased, multiple physicians, or specialists, are required to address many different conditions.

These specialties can be seen as silos of care, each standing separate from the other. Each physician has a specific role in your healthcare, whether you go to a cardiologist for your heart, or to an endocrinologist for your diabetes, or to a primary care physician for your general needs. Ideally, the primary care provider helps you understand input from specialists and oversees integration of recommendations and prescriptions into an overall plan. Unfortunately, in the current healthcare system, it is not possible for one provider to oversee the *whole* you.

As a physician, I see this as a problem. I also experience it as an issue when I am a patient. When I seek care, I want a provider who is overseeing my total health and teaching me how to achieve it. Only after I embraced the definition of physician as teacher did I understand the full dimension of the profession. You see, I as a physician cannot be part of the healing process without teaching the patient and their loved ones about illness, the process of healing, and self-care aimed toward lasting health.

The Cost of the Healthcare System

What is our current healthcare crisis costing us?

The Centers for Medicare and Medicaid Services, a division of Health and Human Services, found in 2015 that, nationwide, healthcare was costing us $3.2 trillion.[1] In the United States, we are spending one out of every five dollars on healthcare. It is projected that we will be bankrupting our healthcare system by the year 2025 if we continue this same trajectory.

We know that from the years 2000 to 2014, according to the Department of Health and Human Services, our spending on healthcare more than doubled. At present, this amount represents 17.5 percent of the gross domestic product.

Would you agree that this is not sustainable?

---

1   cms.gov/Research-Statistics-Data-and-Systems/Statistics-Trends-and-Reports/NationalHealthExpendData/Downloads/highlights.pdf

The high cost of treatment combined with increasing rates of disease places a burden on our resources that we cannot sustain.

What Are You Getting Out of It?

I want to challenge you, as my reader, to think about what you are getting out of this system. It is a system that is fallible, and it is unsustainable because of the increasing costs and the growth of health problems in our country.

I would contend that despite our modern healthcare system, we are getting sicker, as evidenced by increasing chronic disease and obesity rates in our country.

Ask yourself:

- Are you receiving what you expect from the current healthcare system?

- Is your current state of health allowing you to thrive, or simply survive, each day?

- Are you satisfied, or do you believe you are worth more?

There are many diseases that have increased in number in the U.S. population. We know from statistics and from reports from the Centers for Disease Control (CDC) and Prevention that heart disease and cancer are killing more people than the next eight leading causes of death combined. This is cause for concern.

Even more concerning is a 2016 study by Johns Hopkins, published in the *British Medical Journal,* indicating the third leading cause of death in the United States is medical error. Medical errors account for more than 250,000 deaths per year in the United States.[2] This is equivalent to four jumbo jets colliding *every week.* It is important to understand medical error is not due to inherently bad doctors. Most errors represent a system problem. This makes medical errors the number three cause of death in our healthcare system.

It seems that our healthcare system should be making us healthy.

However, with all of these indications, is it keeping its promise to you?

If the system were truly providing you with health, wouldn't a reflection of that be an increase in your life expectancy?

Let's compare our life expectancy to other countries around the world, those who share the Earth with us. What do you believe the life expectancy is in the United States, the country with the most advanced healthcare system in the world?

---

2   bmj.com/content/353/bmj.i2139

Wouldn't you expect that it would only be increasing, given the great number of medical advances and discoveries that we make in the health and pharmaceutical industries?

Before I let you know the life expectancy of those who live in the United States, let me first tell you that it is *not* the longest in the world. The citizens of Japan have the longest life expectancy, at eighty-four years. The United States does not even come in among the top ten countries. The life expectancy of the average American is seventy-eight years.[3]

Now think about your friends or relatives who have passed:

- How old were they?
- Did they have a chronic illness?
- Is this acceptable to you?

If our healthcare system is not providing us with longer lives, and statistics of disease burdens continue to rise, is it logical to conclude that our healthcare system cannot meet our expectations?

As I write this, my great-grandmother turned 105 one week ago. When she turned 100, she said "I'm starting over! I want to do something special on every birthday I have from now on. I want to ride a motorcycle on my

---

3   cdc.gov/nchs/fastats/deaths.htm

birthday!" And that is exactly what she has done for the past five years.

I recently saw her on Mother's Day. If you ask her what her secret is, she will not tell you that her doctor or local hospital helped her live this long. In fact, she will tell you that the time she started feeling worse was when she started to see doctors. She was ninety-three years old when she went to her cardiologist and was found to have right coronary artery blockage. A stent was suggested, but the doctor told her that he would not perform the surgery because she was too old.

Without the stent, my great-grandmother has now lived twelve years longer than that know-it-all doctor thought she would. I'm not even sure that *he* is still alive.

I was born when she was sixty-five. My earliest memories of her are of the times when she worked with my great-grandfather in their one-acre garden. She would wear a large sunbonnet and mud boots, and he wore a straw hat as he worked the soil with a hoe.

At every meal that we shared with them, my great-grandmother would announce which vegetables and berries came out of their garden. Everything tasted so much better when it came fresh from their garden! I didn't know at the time how important my great-grandparents' garden would be to me later in my life.

My great-grandmother will tell you that she has always eaten eggs, bacon, and anything from the garden, which, along with God's provision, has provided her with 105 years of life.

A HEALTHCARE SYSTEM BUILT ON SAND

To continue to rely on this fallible healthcare system is like building a beautiful house on sand. It is beautiful on the outside, it appears to serve a purpose, but if the foundation begins to crumble, then it can no longer provide the security we expected.

Where is this system leading us?

We believed that the healthcare system, pharmaceuticals, and physicians, all working together, were meant for good. They were intended to cure us from our illness. Upon closer analysis, however, these foundational structures are crumbling.

The System Itself

The system itself has changed. Hospital systems are one example of this change. From the beginning of civilized history, hospitals were created to care for the acutely ill and severely wounded. Known as *healing centers*, hospital establishment became part of the church's mission. The current hospital system was birthed from church-community sponsorships. The first hospital was set up in 1663 in New York for wounded soldiers and the first incorporated hospital was established in 1751 in Philadelphia, Pennsylvania. These hospitals were locations for those who needed specialized care and lengthy stays to heal.[4]

Now we find large hospitals housing individuals that used to be treated in the home by the physician. While at times this is beneficial, it also is a significant financial burden. To contain costs, regulations now limit length of stay, often at the expense of full healing.

Doctors find themselves absorbed into the hospital system where we had to adapt to the ever-rising burden of chronic disease. Physicians no longer have the time to educate patients and families about healthy lifestyles for long-lasting wellness. Through the influence of Big Pharma, physicians find themselves matching maladies to medications and moving to the next chronic disease.

Big Pharma

Part of the reason that physicians are unable to give a lasting cure is because we are not able to meet your expectations for rapid relief. Many patients rely upon the pharmaceutical industry to cure them.

---

4   Virginia Health Information. "The Beginning of Hospitals." vhi.org/hguide_beginning.asp

Everyone knows that there is a pill for every ill, right?

If you walk in with a symptom, then I can probably find a medication for your particular illness. For that one pill, however, I will also need to prescribe on average an additional four medications to counter the side effects from the initial prescription.

As we discuss later in the book, the availability of some prescription medications may create a false sense of security and lead a patient to believe they are cured. Relying solely on the medication eventually leads one to ignore or abandon lifestyle choices, which in conjunction with the medications, have afforded optimal well-being.

Do you have any guesses how many prescriptions the average American takes?

Do you know, on average, how many prescriptions people your age are prescribed in America?

Let's take a closer look.

Based on 2013 data, I have found:

- For patients ages twenty-six to forty-nine, the average person takes ten prescriptions.

- If you are between the ages of fifty and sixty-four, the average is 19.2 prescriptions.

- If you are between the ages of sixty-five and seventy-nine, the average is 27.3 prescriptions.

- And if you are eighty years old or older, you may take as many as twenty-nine prescriptions.

Combining all these data brings us to the conclusion that the average American takes 12.2 prescriptions! This number of prescriptions is scary. It should be a cause for concern for every American. As a physician, I want to challenge us all to do something different, something better. When you are once given a medication, a doctor will rarely take you off it, so you become a lifetime subscriber to a pharmaceutical. I believe we are better than that, and we can overcome our illnesses in better ways.

The pharmaceutical industry has been very influential through their marketing. If you are watching TV this evening, I want you to count how many pharma commercials you see. They will catch your eye because usually they feature actors who look like ordinary people.

I also want you to count this evening how many times you hear the phrase *ask your doctor if this is the right drug for you.* I bet that ordinarily you wouldn't even notice how often this phrase occurs, but when you pay attention and start counting, you will be amazed.

Pharmaceutical industries have been brilliant marketers.

Why?

Because they go directly to you, the consumer, and they tell *you* to ask your physician what to do. This is called *direct-to-consumer* advertising.

Do you know that the United States is one of only two countries in the world who allow this?

The United States and New Zealand are the only two countries in the world that allow pharmaceutical companies to advertise to you directly.[5]

It's interesting how health has been commercialized. As a physician, this is very concerning. We must wake up and recognize how skillful advertising persuades us and what it costs our health.

Doctors

I went to medical school and began my career to help heal people. Once I was immersed in my education, I found that it was highly influenced by pharmaceutical industries and pharmaceutical reps. During medical training, we are taught not only generic drug names

5   Ventola, C. Lee. "Direct-to-Consumer Pharmaceutical Advertising: Therapeutic or Toxic?" Pharmacy and Therapeutics. 2011. ncbi.nlm.nih.gov/pmc/articles/PMC3278148/

but also brand name drugs for medications that are created and patented by pharmaceutical companies.

There were a great number of visits and luncheons sponsored by drug representatives, which were welcomed by starving medical students. They gave us a lot of pens and other objects that they put their advertisements on. But throughout all this, what I did not find, and I will discuss this later when I talk about my story, is that it did not answer my desire to help heal people.

Since I have been in practice, the workload demands doing more and seeing more patients. This has compromised my doctor-patient relationships to a serious degree. I cannot, in fifteen minutes four times a year, invest the time as a teacher to help fulfill your desire for lasting health.

When, as a doctor, I noticed the cracks in the foundation I was relying on, I recognized it was no longer a safe place for me try to help you. I needed the opportunity to become the teacher that you deserve for lasting health without the outside influences that cause the foundation to crumble.

OUR COMMUNITIES ARE BECOMING SICKER

We have discussed our current healthcare system and how fallible and unsustainable it is. We've talked about how we built the healthcare system on a crumbling foundation, and we've examined the crumbling foundation the current healthcare system is built upon. Let's now discuss the effects of our current healthcare system on the communities in which we live.

Insurance and hospitals are challenged with trying to keep up with the ever-increasing burden of disease. This has a direct effect on you and your community.

The Insurance Situation

When do you use your healthcare insurance?

If you're like most people, your answer is: *When I'm sick.*

Why do we call it *health*care insurance; shouldn't we call it *sick*care insurance?

If it were really healthcare, wouldn't the system and your insurance be designed to help you maintain true health?

This is our expectation. However, as insurance has continued to provide for sickcare, our mindsets have actually come to expect us to be sick. We find that because our system is sick, we and our communities are sick as well.

The sad truth of the healthcare situation is that insurance premiums have increased on average about 25 percent, yet there is a shrinking number of networks. One in five Americans have only one insurer to choose from. Insurance was intended to serve us for good. However, over time it has become a burden to us. Not only have our expectations changed, causing us to have a sick mindset, but also the financial burden of increasing premiums and narrow networks adds to the toll on our health and the health of our communities.

I want to challenge you to think about the concept of insured, self-pay health consumers. Let me explain by using an example. In this example, you have an insurance plan with a high $10,000 deductible, which also provides you with a narrow network of providers.

You develop an illness or condition that requires the attention of a specialist, yet that specialist is not available in your narrow network.

If you are like most, you want to see the best specialist for your need. Because of your narrow network, you are now faced with paying high costs to be seen out of the approved insurance network.

If you are like me, you would pay the price, no matter what. I have been in your shoes when one of my children needed a specialist outside of our network. I decided that my daughter's health was worth it, no matter what the cost. The reality is that cost did not come without a wake of personal financial burden behind it.

In these situations, we are insured, self-pay customers. Even without the specialist scenario, everyone who has a high deductible becomes a self-pay consumer of health until they pay the $10,000, at which point they receive the next tier of benefit from their plan.

Every dollar you spend fulfilling your deductible amount comes from your hard-earned money. You are a smart consumer in many areas. You shop for the best value in a car, groceries, clothes, electronics, and many other tangible items.

Why should shopping for your health be any different?

Let me explain. Perhaps you receive a bill for $3,500 for an MRI done in January, the beginning of your insurance coverage. Your friend, who has the same insurance and deductible, had the same MRI on the same day and place. His bill was only $500.

What was the difference?

The difference is that your friend asked a simple question upon scheduling their MRI.

The question was, "What is your cash price for this MRI?"

The cash price was $500. Your friend decided to spend his sickcare dollars wisely by inquiring about the lowest price. Because he did not file with insurance, he was not given the insurance price tag that you were given.

This also applies to X-rays. Insurance prices for these are hundreds of dollars. In some instances, the cash price is less than $100. It may surprise you to know this also applies to larger items, such as outpatient surgeries and procedures. Even if you never need an X-ray, MRI, or an outpatient procedure or surgery, you are likely taking a pharmaceutical as I discussed in the last chapter. Your pharmacist is under an order not to tell you the cheapest cash price *unless you ask.*

This model empowers you as the insured, self-pay health consumer to decide what a reasonable price is for your care. Don't be shy; speak up and ask!

The Disease Burden

As I stated previously, heart disease and cancer are killing more people than the next eight leading causes of death combined. Consider the many factors that increase risk for heart disease and cancer—obesity, smoking, inactivity, and stress. These are all preventable lifestyle choices that precede developing the disease. Not only do they precede development of heart disease and cancer, but they are also leading contributors to the diabetes crisis affecting our communities.

I was having a conversation with a fellow physician about wellness, and I was challenging him to think about what happens in our system to people with diabetes.

How are we treating people with diabetes differently, compared to as recent as five years ago?

We talked about changes in the recommended treatment strategy from the American Diabetes Association, when the first step of treatment was lifestyle management.

However, in recent years this emphasis on lifestyle alone as the first step of treatment has now been changed to lifestyle plus the prescription, metformin.

I asked, "Why do you think that is?"

My colleague said, "We can easily give you a pill for that because we don't have time to do appropriate lifestyle modification education."

I said "Yes, that is exactly right. And so, what do you get — what are the effects — when we give you a pill for that?"

He said, "It should make my blood sugar levels improve."

I answered, "Well, knowing how medications are metabolized in the body, what else could it cause?"

After a thoughtful pause, he responded, "I wonder what it's doing to my liver?"

I replied, "It's one thing to take a medication when you truly need it, but they were never meant to promote irresponsible, self-destructive behavior."

"Let's think about this," I said. "Imagine that you are your diabetic patient and you say to yourself: *I want to eat a nice, thick hamburger, so I will take two shots of insulin. You know what, I think I want some fries, too. I'll just give myself another shot of insulin.*

"And you behave like this for ten years, until you are fifty pounds heavier. You look at your ten-year-old child beside you; she is watching your behavior and mimicking your relationship with food. Why is it surprising that your ten-year-old is obese and at risk for developing type 2 diabetes? Type 2 diabetes is not an adult disease anymore."

This conversation brings me to my next point, which are the childhood obesity rates in our country.

One of the most sobering statements regarding the severity of the childhood obesity epidemic comes from former Surgeon General Richard Carmona, who stated, "Because of the increasing rates of obesity, unhealthy eating habits, and physical inactivity, we may see the first generation that will be less healthy and have a shorter life expectancy than their parents."

What does the childhood obesity rate look like?

Data from the Centers for Disease Control and Prevention for 2013 to 2014 show the following:

- For children and young adults between the ages of two and nineteen, the obesity rate was an average of 17 percent of patients.

- Between the ages of twelve and nineteen, the average was 20.5 percent.

- By contrast, the average was 13.9 percent in the year 1999 to 2000.[6]

Now, let us consider adult obesity. There are three categories of obesity:

6   Ogden, CL, et al. "Prevalence of obesity among adults and youth: United States, 2011–2014." NCHS data brief, no 219. Hyattsville, MD: National Center for Health Statistics. 2015. surgeongeneral.gov/news/testimony/childobesity03022004. html

1. *Overweight* is defined as a body mass index (BMI) of 25–29.

2. *Obese* is defined as a BMI of 30–40.

3. *Extremely obesity* is defined as a BMI greater than 40.

In the United States, 32.7 percent of adults age twenty and older are overweight, 37.9 percent are obese, and 7.7 percent are extremely obese, based on BMI.[7]

More than one-third of the U.S. population was considered obese in 2014. This has increased from 30.5 percent in 1999–2000.[8]

This should be sobering, and the rate is rising. If these trends continue, by the year 2030, studies suggest 51 percent of the U.S. population will be obese.[9]

This is not without cost. The astounding annual cost of illness related to obesity is greater than $190 billion.[10]

7   Centers for Disease Control and Prevention. "Health E-stats: Prevalence of overweight, obesity, and extreme obesity among adults aged 20 and over: United States, 1960–1962 through 2013–2014" (2016, July). cdc.gov/nchs/data/hestat/obesity_13_14/obesity_adult_13_14.pdf
8   Ogden et al. "Prevalence of obesity." 2015. surgeongeneral.gov
9   Finkelstein, E. A., et al. "Obesity and severe obesity forecasts through 2030." *Am J Prev Med*, 42, 563–570. 2012.
10   Taylor, W. C., et al.). "The healthy weight disparity index: Why we need it to solve the obesity crisis." *Journal of Health Care*

Sadly, this does not have to be. The billions of dollars being spent are for a preventable disease burden that can be improved with appropriate care for body, mind, and spirit. When only dieting is promoted without attention paid to the wellness of mind and spirit, many people fail to maintain weight loss and often regain their weight within five years.[11]

The Size of Hospitals

We have talked about the problems of our healthcare system in this chapter:

- It makes us sicker.
- It costs us more.
- It does not give us what we are expecting—our health.

I want you to think about the size of your local hospital.

Can you remember a time when your local hospital took up less space than it does now?

I believe that a sick community is reflected by the size of its hospital. In other words, the larger the hospital is, the sicker the community is likely to be.

---

for the Poor and Underserved, 26, 1187–1200. 2015.
11   Forman, E. M., et al. "The mind your health project: A randomized controlled trial of an innovative behavioral treatment for obesity." *Obesity*, 21, 1119–1126. 2013.

We need to think about our healthcare system in new and different ways, about how it is *our* health. We need to come up with an approach that enables us to take charge of ourselves in order to take charge of *our* health. You are worth it: your health, your legacy is worth it.

To quote Tommy Thompson, the former Secretary of Health and Human Services, "To stem the epidemic of preventable diseases that threatens too many Americans, we need to move from a healthcare system that treats disease to one that avoids disease through wiser personal choices."[12]

---

12 Pear, R. "Emphasize Disease Prevention, Health Secretary Tells Insurers." *New York Times*. A14. January 22, 2003. nytimes.com/2003/01/22/us/emphasize-disease-prevention-health-secretary-tells-insurers.html

CHAPTER TWO

Our Dependence on Modern Methods

A PILL FOR EVERY ILL

We can all agree that we rely too much on modern approaches for maintaining our health, and one reason is that we have a pill for every ill. It is important to discuss this as we learn more about our system and the changes we can make toward helping ourselves become well.

You Have a Disease

Imagine that you begin experiencing certain symptoms; they could be vague or specific. You might choose to go online and find a website where you can search for information about these symptoms. You will probably find a diagnosis or several options for what your symptoms might mean. Much of the time, however, the website will offer you a specific disease name.

You make an appointment with your doctor. You are anxious before you see her. At the appointment, you tell your doctor that you have the disease you found through your internet research.

No matter what diagnosis you believe you have, your doctor will need to do the appropriate testing to confirm the diagnosis. Many times, the doctor will talk you down off the ledge and reassure you that the symptoms are not the disease the internet told you it is. This brings you peace of mind and likely saves you lots of money.

The fact is your symptoms are just the tip of the iceberg. They really do not explain all that is going on within you. The medical website is reinforcing your sick mindset.

You are telling yourself: *I'm sick, so I must need a pill for that.*

Is the issue truly a disease?

Why don't we begin with exploring the root-cause of the symptom?

The Doctor Has a Specific Pill to Prescribe

If you are sick, you must need a pill, right?

There are pills for everything. We take medications for high blood pressure, diabetes, cholesterol, GI distress, anxiety, pain, and so on. Because we take our pills as ordered, often our symptoms are under control, and we consider ourselves cured. However, I want to challenge you to think about what happens when you forget to take the medication.

If you were truly cured and you stopped taking the medication, then your symptoms would not return, correct?

The following quote comes from the textbook of *Functional Medicine, 2010*: "Physicians (and now patients, as well) are subjected to the disproportionate impact the drug industries ad campaigns have on information about treatment approaches for disease — everything is centered on taking a drug rather than helping patients change behavior."[13]

Remember previously that I discussed that the United States and New Zealand are the only two countries that allow direct-to-consumer advertising of pharmaceuticals?

Now, consider the impact of this on the physician. You, the consumer, require the professional license of

---

13   Jones, D. S., J. S. Bland, and S. Quinn. "What is Functional Medicine?" In *Textbook of Functional Medicine.* Gig Harbor, WA: The Institute for Functional Medicine. 2010. 9.

the doctor to receive the advertised medication. The doctor now has pressures from the pharmaceutical representatives as well as the patient, all day, every day.

This is not what I envisioned my role as a physician to be when I entered medical school. The sad truth is that this is only getting worse.

You Trust the Doctor's Decision

It is a high compliment to me as a physician when the patient says, "You're the doctor. I believe that you know what's best for me."

However, often I see it as unfortunate that patients are not health advocates for themselves or their loved ones. I appreciate that a patient trusts me, but it is your body and you should learn everything you can about your options.

As I mentioned before, in medical school, doctors are ultimately educated in their specialty. Often, doctors who are specialists may not understand how any two or more medications outside of their specialty affect each other or how another medication may be helpful for you in the setting of a large list of existing pharmaceuticals. Therefore, it is very important for you, as the patient, to ask as many questions as you can of the physician.

The time barrier which exists at your visit does not allow you to always have your questions addressed; this only exacerbates the problem. Instead of having a conversation about the symptom you developed since starting the new medication, or considering that symptom may be a side effect of the medication, you are given additional medications to counter the side effects. Thus, your medication list continues to grow.

Why is it that when the physician recommends pharmaceuticals, you are less inclined to ask questions or ask for alternatives?

This goes back to the sick mindset and belief system that every symptom indicates you need (fill-in-the-blank) medication.

On the other hand, if a doctor discusses making lifestyle choices, such as eating better and exercising, rather than considering the need for medications, this is often met with great scoffing on the part of the patient.

How do I know this?

I have worked in the traditional system for almost a decade and I can replay the sick mindset scenario over and over: *Just give me the prescription, and I will be just fine, doc.*

Let's not forget the scenario where the good doctor has to make adjustments to medications based on national guidelines or recommendations. Guidelines do not treat you as an individual or allow your health care to be personalized. While certain parts of them are beneficial, they can jeopardize the autonomy of the doctor-patient relationship. In these circumstances, the doctor is no longer a collaborator for your health; rather, as regulations overtake relationships, they are treated unkindly and often like the enemy. I have been that doctor many times. This is not what I had envisioned since the age seven of what it meant to be a doctor.

CAUSES FOR SELF-DESTRUCTIVE BEHAVIORS

In the previous section, "A Pill for Every Ill," I introduced the idea that using pills to address every ill encourages irresponsible, self-destructive behavior and, in some instances, may become the cause for worse results than the health issue that you originally faced. This is further explored in the following sections.

Fat-Loaded Burgers and Diabetes

In Chapter One, I described a conversation that I had with a colleague. We agreed that in the current system, it's easier to prescribe a pill than to talk to a patient about lifestyle changes. Even though the American Diabetes Association has changed its recommendations to include medications in addition to lifestyle modifications as first-line therapy, I believe that our patients are better off when they take responsibility for their health and take steps to change their habits.

Medications are necessary at times. However, when the long-term use of them encourages irresponsible, self-destructive behavior through the discounting of the importance of lifestyle choices, I wonder what message is being sent.

For example, if the pill or the shot of insulin will control the symptoms, then why can't the patient continue to enjoy sugar, fat-laden foods, and sedentary habits?

A patient who changes their habits is setting an example for their family and friends. Healthy lifestyle changes are beneficial for everyone involved.

Statins and the Body Mass Index

A study that caught my attention examined the effects of cholesterol-lowering medication, comparing the eating habits of statin users and nonusers.[14] This study looked at calorie and fat intake between these two groups. The researchers followed thirty thousand people over a ten-year period and concluded that those

---

14 Sugiyama, T., et al., "Different Time Trends of Caloric and Fat Intake Between Statin Users and Nonusers Among US Adults: Gluttony in the Time of Statins?" *JAMA, Internal Medicine* (April 24, 2014). jamanetwork.com/journals/ jamainternalmedicine/fullarticle/1861769

people who took the cholesterol-lowering medication ate foods with more calories and fat than those who did not take the cholesterol-lowering medication. In fact, the body mass index (BMI) of those taking cholesterol-lowering medication increased faster than the BMIs of those who were not taking the statins.

This study scientifically demonstrates the concept of a pill encouraging irresponsible, self-destructive behavior.

You and Your Legacy

Legacy is defined as "anything handed down from the past as from an ancestor or predecessor."

I want to ask my patients, and you, the reader, "Who is watching you, and what is your lifestyle teaching someone else?"

We pass on to our families those things that we consider to be important. We are defined by our family of origin.

Often, we do things because "This is just how my family has always done it."

This reminds me of the story of a woman who always cut off the end of a roast when it was about to be put into the oven. She was never really sure why she had been taught to do this.

She asked her mother, who said, "Well, that's the way your grandmother always did it."

Then, the woman asked her grandmother, who said, "I cut off the end of the roast because my roasting pan was too small."

Because Grandma had a habit of chopping off the end of the roast, her daughter and then her granddaughter also did. This is such a simple story, but it makes the point that we can affect the legacy of our family for generations.

If I have healthy habits, will my kids and grandkids have good health habits?

Maybe they won't even think about it.

Wouldn't it be nice if my children and grandchildren said "I eat right, I exercise, I take care of myself, because that's just what my family has always done"?

Remember that I mentioned my 105-year-old great-grandmother in the first chapter?

Whether she realized it or not, she was passing on a legacy of gardening and homesteading, and it came down to me. However, I did not realize this until I was in my thirties. Now that I have fully grasped the concept of leaving a health legacy; I am so thankful for all of those hot days that I spent watching her dig in the soil of the garden. She was showing me how to create health.

GENERATIONAL HEALTH

I have painted the picture that our healthcare system is in crisis, that doctors are encouraged to give pills for all ills, and that sometimes these pills support our lifestyle choices that are detrimental to our long-term health. However, you can also choose to begin now to improve your health for yourself and for future generations.

Recognize That You Have a Role in Your Health Legacy

I hope that you are now thinking about whom your lifestyle may be influencing and what kind of legacy you may be leaving. Perhaps you are thinking about how you would like to improve your legacy.

The fact is that no one else but you can run your race or live your life. No one is perfect; we've all made mistakes. However, through those mistakes and challenges, we have learned that *how* we respond is what matters most.

My questions to you would be:

- Are you going to rise from the ashes, step toward a better life, and make something positive out of these mistakes?

- Or are you going to let your mistakes keep you down, defining you and your legacy?

I like to tell my patients, "Don't feel guilty because you have made bad choices; you didn't know better. The fact is that once you do know better, once you are equipped with that knowledge, then you can take action and do better."

Maya Angelou, author and poet, said, "Once you know better, you do better."

You do have a role in your health legacy. You do have a role in what you are passing on to future generations.

I believe that leaving a health legacy is a responsibility that I have to my children and grandchildren (and hopefully great-grandchildren, too).

You're Never Too Old to Start

Maybe you are reading this book and you are thinking that this sounds good, but it is too late to make a change. I want to tell you about a woman named Harriette Thompson. She is ninety-two years old, and she is the oldest woman ever to run a marathon. That is awesome in itself, but what is even more incredible is that she didn't start running marathons until she was seventy-six years old!

I don't know how many of you have ever attempted to run a marathon. I have, and I did not succeed at the age of thirty-eight. What I take away from the story of Harriette Thompson is that it's not too late for me to complete a marathon—perhaps I just started when I was too young.

I hope you take heart and believe that you are never too old to make a change, especially one that will benefit your health outcomes or change your health legacy.

I promised myself that I would run (or walk) that marathon. It may not be until the eighth decade of my life, but I do not consider my past attempt as the only time that I will ever challenge myself to finish a race.

Decide What Your Legacy Will Be

We've all heard the saying by Dr. C. Everett Koop, the former U.S. Surgeon General: "The best prescription is knowledge."[15]

---

15 Stetson, Dana. "The Best Prescription Is Knowledge." hosa. org/emag/articles/chapter_news_jan07_pg3.pdf

We still know that it is not enough to have only knowledge.

So, what do we need to do with our knowledge?

We need to act upon it.

I hope that this book serves you as an excellent part of your knowledge base. The fact is that you must do some additional research yourself, get plugged into those areas of education that interest you, and arm yourself to take action.

Where I am talking about taking action now is in your health legacy and the generations that come after you. You can teach them a better way based on the example of your life, your stories, your education, and your health outcomes.

Dr. Mark Hyman said, "The key to creating health is figuring out the cause of the problem and then providing the right conditions for the body and soul to thrive."[16]

I could not agree more.

---

16 drhyman.com/blog/2013/05/24/the-one-diet-that-can-cure-most-disease-part-ii/

CHAPTER THREE

A Different Way to Be a Doctor

MY CALLING AT AGE SEVEN TO BE A HEALER

I want to share my personal story with you. I think it is important for you to understand where I am coming from, now that you have seen part of my passion for health and healing already unfolding. It is very important to me that you understand who I am, so that you understand the direction we can travel together.

What Did *Healer* Mean?

When you were a child, did your family and teachers ask you what you wanted to be when you grew up?

I don't remember every time that I was asked that, but I have been told by my parents that when I was seven, I told everyone that I wanted to be a doctor. It's interesting to hear this, because the word *doctor* transformed over time to *healer*.

At age seven, I didn't know what *healer* meant, but I did know who a doctor was. That was what I felt my calling was when I was young, and I continued to want to be a doctor as I grew up.

I didn't know any other path to my goal than to be a traditional medical doctor, because that was what was familiar to me in my life and in my family. Becoming a medical doctor was an ambitious goal and a substantial achievement, especially in a family in which only one of my parents had completed college. By pursuing my dream and continuing to learn, I now know what being a healer means.

The Path to Becoming a Medical Doctor

The career path that seemed to fit my calling was to become a traditional medical doctor. So, I went to school, I completed training programs, and I spent thirteen years in education to achieve what I thought was my calling. I chose the route of traditional medical training to earn my medical doctorate.

During these years of education and training, I was fortunate to train with the best. You see, I was accepted at Harvard for the final part of my specialty training.

The story of how this happened still surprises me. I was not always confident in myself, but I was encouraged to apply to several fellowship programs across the country by my mentor.

He said, "Apply to Massachusetts General, too."

I doubtfully said, "Harvard? Really?"

And my mentor replied, "You'll never know if you don't try."

So, I applied. A while later, I received notice that I had an interview. It was a moment in my life when I felt excited yet terrified at the same time.

As I walked onto the campus, I did my best to appear awake (after two hours of sleep) and confident (I could have puked on demand). I had my first interview with the fellowship director and I felt like I bombed it, but I remained calm and confident.

Then, I moved on to the biggest interview of my life. The interview was with the chair of the department—the author of many articles, chapters, and textbooks that I had studied. His office was small and he invited me to sit down. He started with a few questions, and then came the big one, the one question that I had not prepared for.

He asked, "Why do you want to come here?"

This was a seemingly simple question, yet so much depended on it.

In the few endless moments that it took to gather my thoughts, I sat up straighter in my chair, adjusted my posture, squared my shoulders, and with all the courage that my five-foot-two-inch self could muster, I replied, "Because I want to train with the best so I can be the best. That is why I want to come here. You are the best and this is the best place for me to learn."

My most intimidating interview turned out to be one of the best moments of my life. I flew back home and waited for a few short weeks. I had just finished my peanut butter and jelly sandwich—I was not eating with my current health convictions at this time in my life—when the phone rang. It was the fellowship director.

"Carmen, will you come join us in the program?"

"Really? Are you joking?!" I blurted out.

Then, we both laughed, and I said, "Of course, I would love to!"

That was one of the best years of my life. I learned so much about myself and my specialty. I am forever grateful for the opportunity to study at Harvard, which has helped to mold me into the person I am today. It was a major confidence-building experience for me.

At the end of my education, I thought that I had arrived and had become a super-doctor.

But then I began to question myself: *Was I really that good?*

Barriers and Challenges

To give you an idea of what I was going through during those thirteen years of training and school, but without going into too much detail, it suffices to say that there were hours upon hours of training, learning, and practicing.

Despite it all, my life kept rolling on. I married. I began a family. I had one child while I was in training, and then, during my first year after training, I had twins (surprise!). During the year when the twins were born, I was also *boarding*: taking all of the exams necessary to be a board-certified medical doctor.

In the midst of all this, I became aware that I was in a job situation that was not satisfying my professional needs, and I picked up my family and moved to another opportunity. There I became medical director of a pain management department. My burgeoning career meant that I was taking time away from my family.

Was I taking care of my health while I pursued my career?

My general feelings were a reflection of my stressful lifestyle:

- Brain fog during the workday
- Irritable at the end of the day
- Exhausted at the end of the week
- Not sleeping for days at a time

I was highly stressed. I was eating without mindfulness. If you had seen me in my office with a patient or if you had run into me on the street, I would have looked pretty normal. However, as I am sure you can guess, I didn't feel very good.

A HARVARD-TRAINED DOCTOR HAS A HEALTHCARE CRISIS

Now that you know a little bit about my history, you will understand how I stumbled into my own personal healthcare crisis. It seems paradoxical that a super-doctor would have a healthcare crisis. It was a valuable lesson for me. By living through this vulnerable, frightening time, I finally learned how to look after myself, and it enabled me to help my patients go through their health crises, too.

My Crisis

In the previous section, I admitted that my stressful life didn't feel very good. That is really an understatement — actually, I felt like crap!

Who would guess that I had gestational diabetes when I was pregnant with my twins?

Would you guess, if you look at my photo at the back of this book or on my website, that I had once been diagnosed as prediabetic?

I have had my own struggles with weight, but I figured everything was okay because I was surviving, just like everyone else:

- We all come home from work exhausted and irritable.

- We all experience the guilt of not exercising.

- We are all too worn out to follow conversations with our loved ones, because everyone experiences brain fog.

- We all fall asleep while reading aloud in the evening to our kids, grandkids, nieces, and nephews.

Or am I the only person who acts this way?

I simply thought that this way of life was normal. I felt terrible and yet I had to keep going. I had to keep on being super-doctor, super-mom, super-wife, super-daughter, super-fill-in-the-blank, with the many, many hats that I wore every single day.

In fact, I had health warning signs, like dashboard lights that flashed on and off, day after day, week after week, month after month, and even year after year. Finally, I recognized this and decided to approach my health issues head on, just like the buffalo approaches a storm, turning my face toward the storm, not my back.

During the time that passed — the weeks that turned to months that turned to years — my health crisis was not affecting only me, it was starting to affect my son. You see, my son started exhibiting some of the same symptoms that I was experiencing, even though I am thirty years older than he.

My Education About the Crisis

During my health crisis, I found out that my super-doctor abilities were just not enough, even for treating myself. I recognized that I needed more knowledge, and I began to do some personal research. One day, during a lunch break, one of my coworkers showed me a book called *Wheat Belly* by Dr. William Davis. I looked at the cover and bought my own copy of the book.

As I started reading, I realized that it was not only an approach to healthy eating, but perhaps it is would also contain an answer to why I was feeling so poorly. I was in a prediabetic state, and Davis's book addressed my problem. Instead of prescribing medications, he showed how my health could be improved through diet.

This was a foreign concept to me — and I was a doctor. I did not believe that what I put in my mouth made any difference in my body, because during my medical education I was not trained in nutrition or its effects on the human body. Please don't laugh, but when I had this realization, I took the book with me into a closet and put a blanket over my head, because I wanted to hide.

Why?

Because I felt like this was something so different that I wouldn't be accepted if my world of super-doctors knew what I was learning.

Dr. Davis's book opened my mind to new possibilities, gave me a new beginning, and helped my family. From the moment I chose to put into action what I was reading, I made a deal with myself.

I said to myself: *I am going to try this thing . . . what is it, specifically?*

My Decision to Take Action

Imagine me sitting in my closet with my blanket over my head, reading *Wheat Belly.* I didn't even have a flashlight, yet I decided to take action then and there. I had read the introduction and the first chapter of that book, and I made a deal with myself. I was going to take my first step, which turned out to be the first step of my journey to wellness.

You may be curious what was my first step was. I will freely tell you: I decided to change to a gluten-free diet.

Why?

I decided that I wanted to experiment with what the book was talking about for two weeks, because that's about how long it would take me to read the book.

And do you know how I felt after two weeks?

I felt different. After one week, my brain fog was clearing up, my headaches were better, my blood sugars started to level out, and my sleep improved. Added to all this, I must have lost five pounds, and weight loss wasn't even my first goal.

I started to feel better. Along with feeling better, I started wanting to learn more. This little book launched me into a second career of education regarding alternative ways to help my health. I read any article that I could get my hands on, and I listened to podcasts every second that I had. I started listening to audiobooks. I found that there were many, many resources regarding alternative treatments once I simply opened my mind to another way of being healed.

It took more than opening my mind, Dear Reader. As a super-doctor, I had to understand that my years of training simply hadn't provided me with enough knowledge. I needed to know more. Reading one book led to reading another, which led to me enacting another step in my health journey.

Only at that point did I begin to grasp what my calling at age seven had really meant. You see, my purpose to be a healer was transformed, and it is now defined by how I can help you and others discover health and healing. Now, I have found my passion.

Along the way on my health journey, I implemented ideas for myself and then I started educating my family. My little boy became gluten free by his own choice because he had his own experience of improvements in health that he could express at the age of eight. Now, at the age of eleven, he can read labels better than most adults. He has learned how food can truly help him, and he is an educator to others because of this.

I started feeling better. What I recognized was that I had felt bad for so long, I had forgotten what feeling good was like. Maybe you can relate to this. Maybe you can't.

I am certain that I really like feeling better. I really like the feeling of vitality and the return of energy that I had when I started making these small but significant changes in my lifestyle.

A LEGACY OF HEALTH

I want to tell you about when I finally decided that my health was worth my attention. I realized that I could actually achieve my optimum health, as well as do something even better, which is to leave a beneficial health legacy for my family.

An Internal Conflict

Let's go back to the idea of me being a super-doctor. I was taking care of patients every day in the office and I realized, after years of being in practice, that for the majority of my patients, I was not acting in a healing role. I was not fulfilling the role of doctor or healer that my calling at age seven had led me to become. This caused some frustration within me.

I came to recognize some patterns in my practice:

- Many of my patients kept coming back — their symptoms did not seem to improve.

- Many patients grew increasingly dependent on what I could offer as a medical doctor, which was really only my prescription pad.

- Many patients wanted a quick fix.

Yet, what I was experiencing and learning outside those four office walls was something totally different. I felt that I had found a path that led to lasting health and wellness. However, I felt that in my current environment, working within the traditional model of modern medicine, my alternative ideas might not be accepted.

I was living a life of health and wellness in my home. I was treating the root cause of the problems that I had and learning that the symptoms would then take care of themselves. However, in my medical practice, I continued to treat the symptoms of my patients with the usual band-aids. There were days when I simply felt like a hypocrite. I felt as though I was living two lives. I would share a little bit about my self-healing discoveries when people asked me, but I never felt the freedom to show people in my medical practice a different way, a better way.

It was humbling to admit that I, the super-doctor, draped in my super-doctor cape, could not be the savior that so many patients desired when they came to see me. I had to remove the cape, and, when I did, I could feel a new fire burning within me that changed my view about what it meant to be a helper and a healer. I had to ask and answer the *why* question to help me realize that I needed to *unlearn* some of what I had learned back in medical school in order to continue on the path of becoming the healer that you and all my patients need.

In beginning to unlearn, I moved from the realm of practitioner super-doctor to the healer that I was called to be. I changed my mindset, and I decided that feeling bad was not normal.

We are all made to feel vibrant and full of life. Each one of us is a vessel so powerful that it can heal itself with the right tools. I want you to understand that my tools are not the same that you will require, and yours are not the same as the next person.

Health looks different on everyone. It's not always visible, because health starts on the inside. I firmly believe that knowledge is only useful with application. I have been blessed with the gift of learning, but also of teaching. That is the true definition of physician.

I now know my passion and purpose. I know what I was called to do at the age of seven. My passion is health and wellness. My purpose is to help you find and develop the tools that will help you live your vibrant life. I want to help you understand what you are worth and that you are worth it; that you, your family, and your legacy are all worth the healthy and vital you.

Rethinking My Calling as a Healer

What does it mean to be a healer?

To heal is defined as "to make healthy, whole, or sound; restore the health free from ailment."[17]

Health is defined as "the general condition of the body or mind with reference to soundness and vigor, soundness of body or mind, freedom from disease or ailment, vigor, vitality."[18]

I began to ask myself: *Am I restoring the health of my patients in my role as a medical doctor?*

My answer was that I was not. I was not being a healer in my current position in the healthcare system. I had to get back on a track with methods that would help me get back to that seven-year-old girl who had the calling of being a healer.

Why?

---

17 wordreference.com/definition/healing
18 dictionary.com/browse/health

Because it would not only affect my life, my family, and my future, but the many lives that would come across my path for this purpose, and this purpose only.

Furthering My Education

As I mentioned before, once I started gaining interest in alternative health practices — particularly functional medicine — my hunger for learning intensified. I gobbled up articles, books, and podcasts. I started going to education courses on my own time. I didn't care what time it was, it could be on the weekend or at night. Wherever I could get the training and the information is where I went. I discovered a whole new world that was actually an old world, and it's been around a whole lot longer than any of us have.

A few ideas stand out to me about this old world:

- Vitamins are more than alphabet soup.

- Vitamins and minerals obtained from food give people vitality and vigor.

- There isn't a pill for every ill, because there are very few pills available, other than antibiotics.

- People heal their bodies through achieving true health.

- The body is an amazing creation, and if you give it what it needs, it will thrive and heal itself.

Part of what I learned during this process is that the body cannot heal without attending to the effects of stress. I did not have a hobby beyond studying for thirteen years, as I described earlier.

Do you know what I took on as my hobby as an adult?

I started to garden. I had begun to understand the value in growing my own food. I saw my great-grandparents' garden. I realized that gardening was the health legacy they left to me. I garden and I grow my own food to this day.

Have there been highs and lows?

Sure. Life happens. I'm not going to tell you that I am perfect. What I want you to see is that I worked hard to make changes in myself, even though they were not always popular or mainstream.

I decided back in that closet, with a blanket over my head, that I was worth the work to make the changes to have health and vitality. I decided that my family, my legacy, you, and everyone whom I can touch is worth that work. I did it and continue to do it honorably and humbly to this day.

CHAPTER FOUR

You Are Worth Your Health

AN INSIDE-OUT APPROACH

I've shared my story and about how I came to respect myself, find my worth, and invest in my health. Now, I want to share with you how you, too, can embark on a journey of discovering hope, worth, and the value of leaving a health legacy. By the end of this book, I want you to realize not only that you are worth your health, but also that you are worth pursuing it.

Health Begins on a Cellular Level

Imagine an iceberg.

How many of you have seen an iceberg, either up close (yes, I would be jealous of that cruise) or in photos?

The sight of an iceberg brings nothing but sheer awe and a little bit of overwhelm when you realize how much of that iceberg is actually underwater. I want to compare this with your body. I want you to think about the tip of the iceberg as your symptoms, the issues that cause you to go to your physician to ask what can be done. However, now I want you to think of the symptoms as the visible part of the iceberg, while the larger portion under the water is all the changes that have been occurring on the cellular level within your body.

The tip of the iceberg cannot be fully understood without recognizing that the submerged portion exists and exploring it. Only through the deep dive under the surface into root-cause analyses can the tip truly be understood.

When we are able to reach the root cause — the portion below the surface of the iceberg that is causing the symptom to emerge — we will definitely make some strides toward improving our health.

Let's take the example of body shapes. Body shapes are the tip of the iceberg, and they are all around us each day. Think back to your commute today, your coworkers, your family, and friends. If you are like most, you will recall body shapes of all sizes. Sometimes the only ones that make an impact, however, are the large body shapes. It is easy to judge the shell of a person, but with empowered knowledge, I hope to encourage you to look beyond the shell. Looking at the distribution of extra weight gives me clues into the root cause, which is usually a hormonal component.

You may be surprised to know that a lot of overweight people are not overweight primarily because of overeating calories.

For example, what cause do you naturally associate with large buttocks and thighs on a woman?

I think of pregnancy.

Well, some people carry extra weight around their hips, buttocks, and thighs even though they are not pregnant. The predominant hormone that causes this is estrogen. It may be that there are certain stresses or environmental factors in a woman's life that have caused her estrogen to be overactive.

Let's talk about the second type of overweight body shape. Some people accumulate fat around the waist. These people most likely have typical type A personalities or, to put this a different way, these people have their foot on the gas 100 percent of the time and never let up. Yes, I realize I am including myself in this group.

We continue this pattern for several decades and then, when we look in the mirror twenty or thirty years later, we ask ourselves: *Who is that?*

We wonder how this could have happened, how our bodies could have gotten so round while we were always working so hard.

Well, let's think about the root cause. If you are in a state of 100 percent fighting or running all the time, the primary gland that helps you do this is your adrenal glands. These are your fight-or-flight glands, and after a while even they will run down. Your adrenals release cortisol, and cortisol is a steroidal hormone.

Let's think about it a little differently.

Have you ever been given a steroid by your doctor, and then complained that you gained weight when you took it?

It is the most common complaint that I hear when I give a patient a steroidal medication. In this case of overused adrenal glands, you are going and going all the time and you are absolutely giving your body a constant dose of cortisol. The characteristic weight gain pattern is around the midsection.

The third example of excess body weight is a person who looks like they have extra body weight all over. Some say it looks like they're carrying swim floaties all around the body: anywhere you turn there are rolls of stomach fat, hip fat, and back fat. The interesting part about this pattern is that it is usually an indication that the thyroid hormone is involved. The thyroid affects multiple areas throughout the brain and body, which then affects the entire body. This leads to extra fat stores over the entire body.

The final overweight body type I would like to discuss is a person with a larger abdomen. Some people would call this a beer belly. When looking at this from the point of view of the levels of hormones, I am concerned about one thing in particular, and that is insulin. The pattern of body fat on these individuals reveals a hard belly and hard midsection fat. Some say you can thump on it like a drum. The hormone insulin should help us to think about diabetes, which makes us realize that the primary stressor might be carbohydrates or excess sugar. Alcohol is a form of excess sugar, which is why this belly can be caused by too much beer.

One thing to take note of is that one or more of these body types and, thus, hormone problems, may be present. I have just presented them separately to describe how each one works. The fact is that, unless you have the knowledge of how stress relates to hormones in weight gain, it is easy to fall into the belief that you can lose weight by diet and exercise alone. The problem with this belief is that, even with the common approaches to weight loss, including diet program, exercise, surgery, twenty-four-hour access to a gym, and so on, many times it doesn't work because the root causes and the hormone issues don't change.

Inner Health Reflects on the Outside

In our iceberg analogy, we see that issues with hormones at a cellular level are like the enormous portion of an iceberg that is underneath the surface. The tip of the iceberg is like the visible symptoms that reflect the underlying issues. We can turn this analogy around and think about it in a positive manner.

With consistent effort toward health changes, your health will eventually be reflected on the outside through many avenues:

- The way you look
- The way you carry yourself
- The way you smile
- The way your skin and hair and nails look
- The way your eyes glow
- The way you relate to others

In order to achieve the glow of health, we must first change our thought processes. We must look at changing the stresses that we handle every day. Furthermore, we must find out what works for each individual, each of us is unlike any other being on this planet. We must find out what works for you.

Realize that doing anything one time isn't going to have much of an effect, much like one salad doesn't make you healthy and one doughnut doesn't make you fat. As Dr. Hyman, author and doctor to the Clintons, has said, "The key to creating health is figuring out the cause of the problem and providing the right conditions for the body and soul to thrive."[19]

We must make sure that these conditions and all systems on the cellular level function together to culminate in better health that will ultimately be reflected on your outside.

Health Looks Different From What Society Tells Us Is Beautiful

Perhaps you are reading this book and thinking: *I don't need this, I'm thin, I'm healthy.*

However, what is wonderful about reflecting your health from the inside out is that this is going to look different for every one of us. It is really unfortunate that our society tells us we should all look alike. I don't look like anyone around me, and I love that. We are each wonderful, unique beings.

---

19 drhyman.com/blog/2013/05/24/the-one-diet-that-can-cure-most-disease-part-ii/

Let's talk about a phenomenon called *thin on the outside, fat on the inside*. This indicates that, based on many studies we've seen, there is more fat present on a body than muscle. You may look thin on the outside, but in fact you are more fat than muscle. Just because you are thin, my friend, does not always mean that you are healthy.

Dieting will decrease weight but it will not increase muscle mass, which is what is necessary for healthy functioning. In fact, dieting in the traditional sense may make your health worse. Our society tells us that just diet and exercise alone will help us to lose the weight. However, there are so many other components to building and keeping your health.

So, let's look at health indicators such as blood sugar levels, hormone levels, and cholesterol.

You can look great on the outside, but if your sugar is out of range, if your lipids are horrible, then you are still at high risk of disease burden, including heart disease, stroke, and death, even though you meet society's healthy visual ideal. If you are thin but not metabolically healthy, you are at greater risk for disease burden than your overweight but metabolically fit counterpart. I discuss this to let you know that health looks different on every one of us.

GET BEYOND THE IDEA OF PERFECTION

In my recent years of studying new perspectives on health, I have often wondered when it was determined that health and beauty were one and the same. I find this to be far from the truth. The only similarity is that they both come from the inside out.

The Messages from Our Society

We can't turn our heads or enter a store without seeing magazines filled with photographs of slim, beautiful people.

- Who defines beauty?
- Are they the same people who define health?
- Who defines perfection?
- What is the result of our striving to meet society's expectations of slimness?

Our peers have given us the message that we must be thin in order to be attractive. Peers have pressured us, through beauty pageants, billboards, advertisements, and television.

Another kind of image is fitness. Some people lift weights and enter contests to show off shiny, rippling muscles. This is yet another way to create an image of perfection that is very difficult to achieve.

The amount of stress placed on people to meet expectations of perfection means that we are pretty messed up on the cellular level. Stress is the root cause of much of our weight gain. People aren't fat simply because they eat too many fat burgers. We have so many other stressors and environmental issues that are root causes of being overweight and obese.

We need to recognize that health equals beauty only when you are truly healthy, and it may look different from the false message of society.

We are all influenced by our social structures, cultural politics, and economics. I would ask you to remember that there are many different looks that are healthy and beautiful, depending on different cultures. Looks alone do not equal health.

Who Else Has Given Us This Message?

I want to talk about the generations before us. Perhaps you were told by your parents or grandparents that you must succeed at all costs and that you must always strive to be better. I always felt that my life was guided by survival of the fittest because of the path that I chose.

There is pressure passed down by our previous generations, purposely or not, to succeed. Unfortunately, some of you reading this book have been told that you need to look a certain way before you will find a spouse or a life-long companion. That is based only on looks, not health.

We each strive for perfection, but we need to examine why.

IT'S OKAY TO BE OKAY

It is what it is, but it will become what you make it.
~ Popular saying

We all strive for perfection, but the question is for whom, or for whose approval?

This might be stretching all of us a little bit further than is comfortable, but to make progress we need to replace that ideal of perfection with the thought: *I'm okay.*

Taking this a little further, we can tell ourselves: *Today, it is okay for me to be okay.*

Let's talk a little bit more about that for those of you who may be challenged by images of perfection.

Eighty Percent Is Good Enough

The concept that has significantly changed my life and my ability to handle stress is the concept of *80 percent*. I am very much a type A personality. I don't think I could have gotten this far in life if I did not have this personality type, and it has worked well for me, or has it? I know the health risks I have, given my high stress combined with my family history. I had to decide to handle stress differently.

When I ran across the 80 percent rule, I was blown away. It is presented in a very short book called *The 80% Approach* by Dan Sullivan, a book that changed my life.[20]

So, what does 80 percent look like?

Imagine a pie chart. Of that whole circle, 80 percent of that would be four-fifths, clearly a great majority of the chart.

Dan Sullivan suggests that if you strive for perfection, and aim for 100 percent of that entire circle, you may somehow convince yourself the goal is not achievable or feel overwhelmed. If you tell yourself that you cannot stop until everything is perfect, you may never start. However, if you adopt a belief that achieving 80 percent of the goal or activity is *good enough,* you may experience greater success.

Why is this?

Whatever degree of perfection is represented by the remaining 20 percent may take longer to achieve than

---

20   Sullivan, Dan. *The 80% Approach*. Strategic Coach. 2013.

the 80 percent you can do to get most of the job done. Recognizing that it is not worth spending too much more time and energy on the difficult 20 percent is what has changed my life.

Let me emphasize to you: 80 percent is success. The significant point for my life was that I was always striving for 100 percent, and sometimes this caused me to procrastinate. It was usually because I was avoiding the 20 percent that was presenting problems and didn't even need to get done.

Let's think about the 80 percent approach in regards to health. If you always shoot for 100 percent of your perfect health definition, you put more stress on yourself, and the continuum toward poor health continues. Recognize that achieving 80 percent is better than achieving nothing. Don't hold yourself back because you are afraid to try or know you can't hit that magic 100 percent.

I've realized in my life, and I hope you realize, too, that chasing perfection will always be a waste of time. You will soon realize that the 20 percent that you leave behind didn't make that much of a difference, anyway. Spend the extra time you have gained, by not pursuing the elusive 20 percent, but on something that will benefit your health. Simply reducing my stress by 20 percent helped my life and my health significantly.

Accept Where You Are and Love Yourself

Think about the last time you walked into a gym. Think about the people you saw. When I went to the gym this week, I saw the weightlifters, the people who are in good shape, and the larger, overweight people.

Can you guess which group of people I want to help and cheer on in each step of their path toward fitness?

I feel compelled to cheer for the people who are overweight because it takes courage and emotional strength to walk into the door of that gym when you are overweight. What I see in these individuals is that they have accepted where they are, and they are taking steps toward their health.

Why do so many of us avoid the gym?

Because we are not in good shape in the first place.

I think it is sad that our society has turned gyms into social meeting places. There are people who really need a gym to help them achieve their new lifestyles. I would challenge you, the next time you are in a gym, to encourage the overweight person who had more drive to walk into the gym that day than you did. You don't know how much it will help them to have the courage to return the next day, and the next day after that.

If you love something, you will take care of it, right?

Understand that growth and change take time. You have to nurture them. I would challenge you to choose to love yourself at every step along the way; don't wait until you are perfect.

Because, guess what?

You never will be your absolute ideal. I promise you that by taking your new health journey, your definition of perfection will change.

When you learn something, do something. Don't wait until you reach your goal to be proud of yourself. Be proud of each step you take toward reaching that goal.

Take Action and Shift Your Own Health Legacy

It is health that is real wealth
and not pieces of gold and silver.
~ Mahatma Gandhi

I challenge you to accept where you are and love yourself for a while and then take action. Only you can shift your own health as well as your health legacy. No one else can make this decision for you. These are your steps to take on your path. People may join you along the way to help or to encourage you, just as you help and encourage others, but this is still your journey to walk. This is your investment. This is your life.

Are you investing in tin cans or gold?

I like this quote from Wayne Dyer, author and inspirational speaker: "Be miserable or motivate yourself."

A motivational quote that has inspired me is, "It is never too late to be what you might have been."

CHAPTER FIVE

Taking Responsibility for Our Own Health

ARE YOU COMPLACENT?

Yes, it's okay to be okay. Now, we must move on to taking control and responsibility for our individual health. To do this, we must reach beyond the modern paternalistic approach that our healthcare system has forced us into. We're going to learn what it looks like to envision our future healthy self and how to reach our vision.

"I Feel Fine"

As you went about your business today, did anyone ask you, "How are you?"

I want you to think about what your answer was. I've become very mindful of this in my own life.

I am trying to not simply answer, "I'm fine! How are you?"

Has *fine* come to mean the same as *mediocre?*

Or do we want *fine* to actually mean what it should mean, which is *healthy and well.* I've come to be mindful of answering this question because people will take a second glance or a second listen when I am honest.

I might be the only person who says, "I'm kind of tired."

I would challenge you to evaluate yourself and your answer to that ordinary question:

- Are you well rested in the morning?
- How many times did you hit snooze on the alarm clock?
- Do you have energy throughout your day?
- Do you have an afternoon low?

If you have made it this far in the book, I hope you realize this is not the definition of fine that you deserve. I want you to be sure that you are not confusing complacency with contentment.

Complacency is the moment when you respond to the person: "Fine, I'm fine."

Complacency is accepting that there are no alternatives and that you will never change. Complacency looks like you are just surviving. Understand the value of moving beyond complacency into contentment.

Contentment comes when you truly step into your purpose and know that you are where you need to be. Contentment is an all-encompassing objective of being well, being healthy. Contentment moves you from simply surviving to thriving!

What's It Going to Take for You to Feel Better?

Are you complacent?

Or are you truly content?

So, what's it gonna take for you to feel better?

Are you going to be one of those people who waits until the bad news gets dropped on your head by a healthcare provider?

Please understand that you don't have to end up sick in the hospital or on twenty medications before you are able to think about feeling well.

Please consider deeply how you would answer these questions:

- Wouldn't it be nice to have the energy to play with your kids after work, and to do the things you love, your hobbies and social gatherings, with energy and gusto?

- What about waking up refreshed before the alarm clock goes off?

- If you have ever experienced this, it's is a great feeling, isn't it?

- What will it take for you to take the steps to begin feeling your best?

Can You Envision Feeling Your Best?

I want you to go back to my story from earlier in the book and remember that there is a period of time when fine may be simply *okay*. At the time, I didn't know anything different, and I had forgotten what good health felt like. Maybe you are at that point, as well.

Remember that when we know better, we do better. A turning point for me was when I started envisioning feeling my best. I knew I had to keep that vision in mind when things got a little tough and rough so that I could continue on my health journey. Maybe you are not on your health journey yet, but maybe you are resolving to begin.

Do you have a firm vision of your best self, living freely and healthfully?

Along my journey I have had many successes and many fallbacks, because I am only human. However, with each step forward that I take, I redefine what is my best. I look back and I see the *fine* person that I used to be, but I also reevaluate and see my best that is yet to come.

Envision you at your best.

What are the barriers you see between you as you are now and that version of yourself?

BEYOND DIET AND EXERCISE

As you consider the barriers to your vision of your best self, identify specific reasons you have not been able to move beyond them. I would challenge you that perhaps you have yet to find the correct tools.

So much emphasis is placed on diet and exercise; however, in reality, this is only a portion of the equation for health and wellness. Diet—aside from containing the word *die*—implies restriction and misery will follow. Approaching the equation from the 80/20 rule, efforts should be focused on the 80 percent, which is nutrition.

When you give the body what it needs, it will thrive. When you begin to view food in this light, every choice you make about eating will be reflective. Exercise is necessary; however, it is false to believe that one can exercise to eat whatever one wants. Sometimes, the best exercise is simply the exercise you know you will do. Some is better than none. We must strive for balance.

Science at the Cellular Level

Earlier in this book, I introduced the analogy of an iceberg, and I will remind you that the majority of the iceberg is not what we see, but is below the surface of the water. When we think of this as our health, remember that the tip of the iceberg is simply the symptom of the underlying condition. Recall that it was the submerged portion of the iceberg that sank the *Titanic*.

Another way I like to describe this is with roots. We must go to the root cause of our symptoms, which is not always visible. We do not always understand or feel all of the cellular processes that are occurring. However, when one cellular process affects the next, and so on, it will ultimately end up as a symptom that you will notice, a symptom that may have taken years to develop. One symptom can lead to other symptoms that are even stronger and demand more attention.

It is important that we respect the body's intricacies at the cellular and biochemical level. Each process in the body is interwoven with other systems. I think of these systems like gears in a clock. One cog-wheel will help the next wheel run smoothly, which will help the arm of the clock move, which will help the second hand to move — second, by second, by second. If one of these cog-wheels is misaligned or one tooth breaks, the whole clock is affected.

The same is true for your body down to your biochemical cellular processes. In the same way the negative symptoms were formed, healing can occur. Identify the root cause, work toward that end, and your clock will eventually run like new.

Mindfulness and De-stressing

We know that long-term chronic stress creates all kinds of health problems.

Why?

Stress changes the wiring in our nervous system, and hormones react as if we are in a constant state of stress. When the body is in this constant state, it will have a hard time distinguishing whether it is hungry, tired, emotional, anxious, and so on. This is because the signals are not being sent out correctly. So, the body sends out signals that say, *eat more, sleep less,* which can, after a while, lead to anxiety or perhaps depression, or emotional states such as anger.

It's time to push reset. It's time to turn that system off. Consider taking a step back; taking a few intentional and slow, deep breaths; and simply slowing down, however difficult that is to do in our society. It seems that it is urgent for us to survive in a very competitive world.

I am not really a stop-and-smell-the-roses kind of person because of the way I have been trained and the career path I chose, but the more birthdays I have, the more I recognize that it's important to stop and smell the roses. Recognize that in order to fully appreciate the rose, you need to not only look at the rose, but also feel the rose, smell the rose, and touch the rose.

Your own life is no different from the rose. You deserve the time to appreciate your life, to take a break, and to reset your mind. When you understand the difference between surviving and thriving, you will be able to reach closer to your best self that you have envisioned.

I love this quote by author and health coach Sid Garza-Hillman: "Caring for the mind is as important and crucial as caring for the body; in fact, one cannot be healthy without the other."[21]

Recognizing or Discovering Your Higher Calling

I want to take you back to my story. When I was seven years old, I told anyone who asked that I wanted to

---

21 Garza-Hillman, Sid. *Approaching the Natural: A Health Manifesto.* Roundtree Press. 2013.

be a doctor when I grew up. I didn't quite know what that meant until many, many decades later. Now, I understand what my higher calling is, and that is to be a healer and an educator.

I ask you and all my patients:

- What is your body saying *no* to?
- What is your higher calling?
- What is your purpose, your passion?
- Are you doing what makes you thrive in life, or is something in your way?

I love this joke by the comedian and television host Steve Harvey: "Your career is what you are paid for; your calling is what you are made for."

Another very poignant quote comes from Sister Ita Ford: "I hope you come to find that which gives life a deeper meaning for you. Something worth living for, maybe even worth dying for. Something that energizes you, enthuses you, and enables you to keep moving ahead. I can't tell you what it might be, that's for you to find, to choose, to love. I can just encourage you to start looking and support you in the search."[22]

Dear Reader, I echo Sister Ford's feelings. I can't tell you what to do, but I can encourage you to envision

---

22 lovingjustwise.com/ita's_words.htm

your best self. And I will definitely support you in your journey.

INVEST IN YOUR OWN HEALTH

Now that you have envisioned your best self, what tools are you going to use to get there?

Your investment is required. Investing in your own health is required in order to leave behind that legacy that you have dreamed of.

What Is Your Health Worth?

Let's face it: we all invest in what is important to us. I can tell you what is important to you if you let me look at your bank account and your bank statement. The fact is that a person will invest his or her money in the areas of life that reflect their values.

You will spend money on a new car, a new boat, or a new house, yet you don't invest in yourself.

Why do you not believe you are worth it?

What is your health worth, so that you can enjoy that new car, that new boat, and the thriving self that you are meant to be?

How many of you have ever said, "I don't have time?"

I'm going to be frank with you. The saying *I don't have time* is simply the grown-up version of *The dog ate my homework*. I think we are all better than that.

Charlie Chaplin said it best:

> As I began to love myself, I freed myself from anything that is no good for my health. Food, people, things, situations, and everything that drew me down and away from myself. At first, I called this attitude a healthy egotism. Today I know that it is love of oneself.[23]

Your health is definitely worth your investment so that you may leave this to your children and grandchildren as your legacy. However, you must first begin with loving yourself.

Who Does It Impact?

Who do you think is watching you?

Everyone has a circle of influence and is making an impact on others, whether it is on your children or your friends or even your pets. Be aware of who is watching you and what you are teaching them with your actions. This is why integrity is so important.

---

23 wolfgangzeitler.de/CharlieChaplin_As_I_began_to_love_myself.pdf

I cannot describe to you the unexpected number of people who have told me I have taught them about health. There are people who will silently watch you, and when you've made an impact on them that they can see and feel, they may one day tell you about it. With every action you take, every choice you make, please recognize it will affect not only you, but it will definitely affect others around you. I will offer you the story of my children.

My oldest child was about eight years old when he told me "Mom, you were right."

Now, who doesn't love to hear that from their child?

At that time, for about a year, I had been changing my diet, and my home is a home of education. I'm not going to tell you what to eat; instead I am going to educate you about why Mommy buys what she does and why she doesn't buy those other things anymore.

One evening my son came down the stairs and said, "Mom, you were right."

I said, "Yes, but what was I right about?"

He said, "That pizza I ate today gave me a headache. You remember? You told me that one of those things that gluten could do to me was give me headaches. I think that's right."

I said "Oh, really? Well, now what are you going to do?"

He said, "I will never eat gluten again, Mom."

That eight-year-old boy is now eleven years old and he has not touched gluten foods since. All that first year, he was watching, listening, and learning while I changed the family's diet.

I would also like to offer a quote by author James Baldwin: "Children have never been very good at listening to the elders, but they have never failed to imitate them."

What Legacy Do You Want to Leave?

I want you to consider:

- What health legacy will you leave?
- How do you want to be remembered?
- How do you want your footsteps to be followed?
- As we have discussed before, do you want to be part of a generation whose children live shorter lives?
- Do you want to be part of the solution for healthy lives for our children?

I revisit this question multiple times throughout the month or with any decision that I'm making: *Will this have the impact that I wish to create?*

And if the answer is that it doesn't have a healthful, valuable impact, then I say no to that direction.

Alexander Rose, a seventeenth-century scholar and bishop, said, "Build something that outlives you," and I truly live by this quote.

I also admire this quote from St. Catherine of Siena: "Be who you were created to be and you will set the world on fire."

Conclusion

Consider your health. Consider your worth. You deserve a healthy life. Your health is worth all you can do, for yourself and to leave a lasting legacy to your children, your grandchildren, and other important people in your life.

This is your time to say, "I am important enough to care for my health, and what I am doing may not be working for me. It is time for a change. I am worth that change."

I want you to go back and read that statement again, Dear Reader, and then I want you to close your eyes for just a moment. I want you imagine your best self three years from now. I want you to imagine not only what you look like, but, more importantly, what you feel like. I want you to imagine what you have accomplished and what you are going to accomplish. Now, open your eyes and decide what steps you are going to take next. Understand, Dear Reader, that the best is yet to come; you need only to take the first step.

Remember, I have been in your shoes.

I myself have had to make the decision to take the first step to do something different, to make choices that are not popular in my world as a doctor:

- I had to define my best self and envision her happy and thriving.

- I had to take steps to align my career with my calling so my purpose in life is fulfilled.

- I had to recognize all this will leave a positive healthy legacy for my children and all of those with whom I am privileged to journey.

No matter the cost, no matter the pain, no matter how great the challenge, I will wholeheartedly tell you that I would do it all again. For you. For our future generations.

I want to encourage you now to find a friend or mentor, someone who understands health and wellness as I have defined it in this book, and ask them to help you start on a new path. If you choose me as your partner in health, I invite you to get in touch with me or my office staff and we will be glad to talk with you about your new journey and how we might work in partnership to pursue it.

I love this quote by Einstein: "We cannot solve our problems with the same thinking we used when we created them."

We also cannot solve our problems with the same *life choices* we made when we created them. I think you understand this better now, after reading my book.

Do not wait. Do not hesitate to take action for your best self. We are not guaranteed that there will be a tomorrow—you can decide to start your new life journey today.

Next Steps

I would love to continue my health journey with you. You can visit my website 360living.today or email my team at 360careteam@360living.today. As a thank-you for reading this book, I invite you to contact us for a discounted first visit with me. Please contact us and we will send you the necessary information.

You can connect with 360 Living on Facebook, Twitter, Pinterest, and Instagram.

I so look forward to hearing from you and I hope to meet you soon.

Until then, always remember to exhale.

Carmen Keith, MD
Founder and Medical Director
360 Living

About the Author

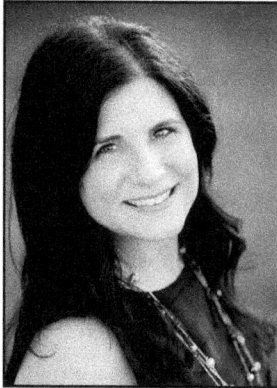

Carmen Keith is a medical doctor and the founder of 360 Living. Dr. Keith received training from the very best teachers in the field of modern medicine in pursuit of her lifelong goal of helping people. Her passion has always been to provide new avenues to health. However, she has discovered that it is not enough to be healthy — the ultimate goal is to be well. In her quest to discover answers for herself, she stepped outside what modern medicine defines as treatment and into methods from days gone by, when doctors looked for answers to treat the whole individual: body, mind, and spirit. On this journey, she discovered she could no longer settle for the status quo or keep the information to herself.

Dr. Keith has found the tools that work for her on her journey to health and wellness. Her passion is to help others discover the same. Dr. Keith firmly believes that each person deserves a healthy life and the opportunity to leave a lasting wellness legacy to future generations. Everyone must make a choice about health.

Are you ready to make a change and choose to live 360?

For more information, please visit 360living.today, or contact 360careteam@360living.today.